1

Table of Contents

Insulin Resistance, also known as impaired insulin sensitivity, happens when cells in your muscles, fat and liver don't respond as they should to insulin, a hormone your pancreas makes that's essential for life and regulating blood glucose (sugar) levels. Insulin resistance can be temporary or chronic and is treatable in some cases.

Under normal circumstances, insulin functions in the following steps:

- Your body breaks down the food you eat into glucose (sugar), which is your body's main source of energy.
- Glucose enters your bloodstream, which signals your pancreas to release insulin.
- Insulin helps glucose in your blood enter your muscle, fat and liver cells so they can use it for energy or store it for later use.
- When glucose enters your cells and the levels in your bloodstream decrease, it signals your pancreas to stop producing insulin.

For several reasons, your muscle, fat and liver cells can respond inappropriately to insulin, which means they can't efficiently take up glucose from your blood or store it. This is insulin resistance. As a result, your pancreas makes more insulin to try to overcome your increasing blood glucose levels. This is called hyperinsulinemia.

As long as your pancreas can make enough insulin to overcome your cells' weak response to insulin, your blood sugar levels will stay in a healthy range. If your cells become too resistant to insulin, it leads to elevated blood glucose levels (hyperglycemia), which, over time, leads to prediabetes and Type 2 diabetes.

In addition to Type 2 diabetes, insulin resistance is associated with several other conditions,

BREAKFAST

1. Curry Vegetable Soup

Prep Time: 35 Minutes

Cook Time: 45 Minutes

Servings: 2

Ingredients

- 2 large carrots chopped or sliced
- 2 large celery stalks chopped
- 1 medium onion chopped
- 1 large sweet potato chopped
- 2 stems broccoli peeled and sliced
- 1 cup green beans cut into 1" pieces
- 2 medium zucchini sliced
- 1 tsp dried oregano
- 1 1/2 tsp dried basil
- 1/2 tsp ground black pepper
- 1 tbsp curry powder to taste

- 2 tbsp maple syrup
- 4 cups low-sodium vegetable broth
- 1/2 cup cooked chickpeas

Instructions

1. In a large pot, heat 1/4 cup of vegetable broth on medium-high heat and add carrots, celery, onion and sauté for 5 minutes.
2. Add sweet potato and broccoli stems and sauté for another 5 minutes.
3. Add oregano, basil, black pepper, curry powder and stir for one minute.
4. Add the vegetable broth, maple syrup, green beans, zucchini, and chickpeas. Bring the soup to a gentle boil and then reduce heat to simmer.
5. Simmer for 20 minutes or until the potatoes are tender.
6. Add another ½ cup of chickpeas if you wish. Instead of chickpeas add your favorite cooked beans.

2. Sweet Potato Bean Tots with Pineapple Tomato Salsa

Prep Time: 15 Minutes

Cook Time: 20 Minutes

Servings: 2

Ingredients

- 1 large sweet potato
- 1 cup canned, low-sodium black beans rinsed & dried
- 1/2 tsp ground cumin
- 1/2 tsp black pepper
- 1/2 tsp garlic powder
- 1 medium onion chopped & divided
- 1 tbsp nutiritional yeast
- 2 cups canned, low-sodium diced tomatoes drained
- 2 green onions chopped
- 1 cup pineapples
- 4 cups baby spinach
- 2 slices 1/2" pineapple

Instructions

1. Preheat the oven to Bake at 400°F. Prepare a baking sheet with parchment paper or silicone mat.
2. Bake the sweet potato in the oven for 30 minutes or until cooked. Once cooked, let cool to handle and scoop out the potato. Set aside.*
3. Sauté the onion, in a little amount of water or low-sodium broth, over medium-high heat for 5 minutes or under soft.
4. In a large bowl, mash together the potato, beans, cumin, black pepper, garlic powder, sautéed onion, and nutritional yeast. Form the mixture into small tots and place on the prepared baking sheet. (Makes 14 to 16). Bake for 30 minutes.
5. In a food processor, pulse the drained tomatoes, green onions, and pineapple chunks a few times so that the salsa is chunky.
6. Serve the tots on a bed of baby spinach and slice of pineapple along with the pineapple tomato salsa
7. Alternately, you can peel the sweet potato and steam it in a steamer until soft. Once cooked, mash the potato and set aside. Add your favorite spice to the tot mixture.

3. Breakfast Sunshine Fruit Bowl

Prep Time: 15 Minutes

Cook Time: 20 Minutes

Servings: 1

Ingredients

- 1 cup Boston lettuce chopped
- 1 cup spinach chopped
- 1/8 large papaya peeled, seeds removed, and cut into chunks
- 2 small oranges (or 1 large orange) peeled & sliced
- 1 mango peeled, pit removed and cut into thick slices
- 1 green kiwi peeled & sliced
- 1 cup pineapple cut into spears
- 1/4 dragon fruit peeled & sliced
- 1 tsp ground flaxseed

Instructions

1. In a small blender place 1 orange, ½ mango and ¼ cup pineapple. Blend until smooth. Set aside and use as dressing for the fruit bowl.
2. In a serving bowl place the lettuce and spinach.
3. In the bowl arrange the fruit, papaya, slices of 1 orange, remaining mango slices, kiwi slices, remaining pineapple spears, and dragon fruit slices.
4. Pour fruit dressing over the fruit and sprinkle with flaxseed.
5. Mix the whole bowl just before eating.

4. Creamy Broccoli Soup

Prep Time: 15 Minutes

Cook Time: 45 Minutes

Servings: 2

Ingredients

- 4 cup Low-Sodium Vegetable Broth
- 1 1/2 cup Onion
- 2 tsp Fresh Garlic
- 1 1/2 cup Red Bell Pepper
- 2 cup Russet Potato with skin on
- 2 cup Parsnips
- 4 cup Broccoli Florets
- 1 cup Unsweetened Almond Milk
- 1/4 cup Nutritional Yeast
- 1/4 tsp Cayenne Pepper
- 1/2 tsp Black Pepper

Instructions

1. In a large pot, heat ¼ cup of vegetable broth at medium-high heat, and then add the diced onion and minced garlic. Sauté, stirring frequently, for 3 to 5

minutes or until the onion is softened. As the broth evaporates, continue adding more, a couple of tablespoons at a time – just enough to barely cover the bottom of the pot and prevent the onions and garlic from sticking.

2. Add the diced red pepper and sauté for another minute or two.

3. Add the remaining broth, along with the diced potato and parsnips. Bring to a boil, then adjust the heat to low. Simmer the vegetables in the broth for 10 minutes, stirring occasionally.

4. Add the broccoli to the pot, and continue simmering for another 10 minutes. Add an additional cup or two of water if necessary, to keep all the vegetables covered in liquid.

5. Check to make sure the potatoes and parsnips are soft by pressing the tip of a sharp knife into one piece. If the blade slides in easily, the vegetables are ready. If not, continue simmering for a few more minutes and check again.

6. Turn off the heat under the pot. Stir in the plain almond milk, nutritional yeast, cayenne pepper, and black pepper.

7. Using an immersion blender (stick blender), or working in batches using a regular kitchen blender, blend the soup until smooth. You may choose to leave the soup slightly chunky, if you prefer.

8. Pro tip: The soup will be very hot, so work carefully and watch for splashes. If you're using a regular kitchen blender, place the blender container in the sink, and then pour the soup into it from there, to help prevent spilling and splashing. Always pour away from you rather than toward yourself.

9. Taste and adjust the seasoning to your liking, if you wish. Serve immediately and enjoy!

5. Kale Potato Salad

Prep Time: 15 Minutes

Cook Time: 25 Minutes

Servings: 2

Ingredients

- 2 cup Red Potatoes
- 4 cup Kale
- 1 cup Low-Sodium Black Beans
- 6 oz Firm Tofu
- 1 cup Tomatoes
- 2 tbsp Capers
- 1/3 cup Red Wine Vinegar
- 1/4 tsp Ground Black Pepper

Instructions

1. Bring a medium pot of water to a boil, and simmer the cubed potatoes for about 10-15 minutes, or until soft enough to pierce easily with the point of a knife. Note

that the smaller you dice the potatoes, the more quickly they'll cook.

2. Drain the potatoes, and if they're already quite soft, you may want to rinse them in cold water to prevent them from cooking any further. Set aside.

3. In a large bowl, combine the chopped kale, crumbled tofu, black beans, chopped tomatoes, and capers.

4. Drizzle the salad with your red wine vinegar, and then sprinkle with ground black pepper.

5. Toss everything together, then serve and enjoy.

6. Apple Broccoli Wild Rice

Prep Time: 15 Minutes

Cook Time: 1 hrs

Servings: 4

Ingredients

- 1 1/2 cup Uncooked Wild Rice
- 1/2 cup Sweetened Dried Cranberries
- 2 3/4 cup Low-Sodium Vegetable Broth
- 2 1/4 cup Fresh Apple Juice
- 1/4 tsp Dried Oregano
- 1/4 tsp Ground Black Pepper
- 1/4 tsp Dried Thyme
- 1 Medium Granny Smith Apple
- 3 Cloves Garlic
- 1/4 cup Raw Pecans
- 1/4 tsp Nutmeg
- 4 cup Broccoli

Instructions

1. In a saucepan, combine 1½ cups wild rice, ½ cup dried cranberries, 2½ cups vegetable broth, 2¼ cups

fresh apple juice, ¼ tsp dried oregano, ¼ tsp black pepper and ¼ tsp dried thyme. Bring to a boil, then reduce the heat to low. Allow the rice to simmer, partially covered and stirring occasionally, for about 55 minutes until the liquid has been absorbed, or until the rice is cooked to your liking.

2. About 10 minutes before the rice is ready, core and dice the apple.

3. Steam the chopped broccoli florets in a steamer for about 5 minutes, or until softened and vibrant in color.

4. In a large frying pan or sauté pan, heat an additional ¼ cup of vegetable broth until hot. Add the diced apple, and stir for 3 minutes. Next, add the minced garlic and chopped pecans. Sprinkle with ¼ tsp nutmeg and stir for a few minutes more.

5. Add the cooked wild rice and steamed broccoli to the apple mixture and stir well.

6. Serve while hot.

7. Stuffed Breakfast Potato Boat

Prep Time: 15 Minutes

Cook Time: 45 Minutes

Servings: 4

Ingredients

- 1 Medium Sweet Potato (about 2 cups)
- 1/2 cup Onion
- 2 Cloves Garlic
- 1 cup Broccoli
- 1 cup Bell Pepper
- 1 cup Mushrooms
- 2 cup Spinach
- 1 tbsp Ground Flaxseed

Instructions

1. Preheat the oven to 425°F. Pierce the sweet potato several times with the tines of a fork. Bake it (whole) on a lined baking sheet until the tip of a knife penetrates the skin easily, about 45-50 minutes.

2. Meanwhile, heat a small amount of water in a frying pan or sauté pan, and then add the diced onions. Sauté for 5 minutes, until the onions soften.

3. Add the minced garlic and sauté for 3 minutes until fragrant.

4. Next add the broccoli florets to give them a head start over the more tender vegetables. After a few minutes, add the diced bell pepper. Finally add the sliced mushrooms, and cook for a total of about 10 minutes over low heat, stirring occasionally, until the vegetables are tender.

5. Turn off the heat and stir in the spinach and ground flaxseed.

6. Cut the sweet potato in half and lightly mash it with a fork.

7. Spoon the sautéed vegetables on top each potato half, and enjoy!

8. Clementine Cranberry Oats

Prep Time: 15 Minutes

Cook Time: 10 Minutes

Servings: 5

Ingredients

- 1/3 cup Rolled Oats
- 1 Orange (juiced), plus enough water to reach 1 cup of liquid
- 1/2 cup Cranberries
- 2 cup Baby Spinach
- 1/2 tsp Cinnamon
- 1 scoop Amla Green
- 1 tsp Ground Flaxseed
- 1 Banana
- 1 Clementine
- 1/2 cup Unsweetened Plant-Based Milk
- 1 tsp Orange Zest

Instructions

1. If you'd like to add orange zest to your dish, zest the orange first, until you have 1 tsp of zest.
2. Squeeze the juice from your orange into a liquid measuring cup. Add water to the juice until you have a total of 1 cup of liquid.
3. In a small saucepan, bring your cup of orange juice and water to a boil. Add the rolled oats and reduce the heat to low, simmering while you stir frequently, for 8-10 minutes, or until the liquid is mostly absorbed.
4. Add the cranberries and chopped baby spinach to the saucepan and stir them in. Cook for another few minutes, until the spinach wilts.
5. Turn off the heat and stir in the cinnamon, ground flaxseed, and Amla Green.
6. Transfer the oat mixture to a serving bowl.
7. Top with the sliced banana and clementine slices.
8. Pour the plant-based milk over the oats, and add the orange zest if you wish.
9. Serve and enjoy!

9. Caulifornia Car-Bowl-Hydrate

Prep Time: 20 Minutes

Cook Time: 10 Minutes

Servings: 5

Ingredients

- 1 cup Cauliflower Rice
- 1 cup Broccoli, steamed
- 1/2 cup Black beans
- 1/2 cup Zucchini, shredded
- 1/2 cup Carrots, shredded
- 1/2 cup Tomatoes, diced
- 1/2 cup Bean sprouts
- 1/2 cup Corn
- 2 cup spinach
- 1 Lemon, juiced
- 1/2 tsp dill

Instructions

1. Mash chickpeas with a fork so there are no whole chickpeas left and the mixture resembles a canned tuna consistency.

2. Stir in the hummus, dijon mustard, capers, chives, pickles, black pepper and lemon juice and mix until well combined and the mixture begins to stick together. You may have to add a splash of water if it's too dry!

3. Spread rice out evenly onto your nori sheets, then add a layer of chickpea filling and cucumber sticks down the middle.

4. Roll up your sushi tightly, slice up and serve with all your favorite sushi condiments!

5. You can also add other vegetables if desired, such as carrots, purple cabbage, green onion, red bell pepper, or spinach.

10. Apple Blueberry Oat Bake

Prep Time: 20 Minutes

Cook Time: 45 Minutes

Servings: 2

Ingredients

- 1 Casserole Dish

- 1/4 cup steel-cut oats
- 1 1/2 cups oat milk or your favorite non-dairy beverage
- 1/2 cup water
- 1 tsp vanilla extract
- 4 medium apples any kind, chopped
- 1 1/4 cup blueberries fresh, or frozen
- 3 cups baby spinach chopped
- 1 tsp ground cinnamon
- 1/4 tsp nutmeg
- 1 tsp ground flaxseed

Instructions

1. Preheat the oven to Bake at 350°F.

2. In a baking dish or casserole dish combine the oats, oat milk, water and vanilla extract. Set aside and let soak while preparing the other ingredients.

3. Once prepared add the apples, blueberries and spinach to the soaked oats and mix.

4. Sprinkle the cinnamon, nutmeg, flaxseed and mix in.

5. Bake for 45 minutes.

6. Serve fresh from the oven and enjoy with a cup of hot tea!

11. Mushroom Pot Pie

Prep Time: 20 Minutes

Cook Time: 45 Minutes

Servings: 2

Ingredients

- 1 medium white potato peeled & diced
- 2 medium carrots finely chopped
- 1 small onion finely diced
- 1/4 cup shallot sliced
- 5 cloves garlic minced
- 2 oyster mushrooms shredded
- 3 cremini mushrooms chopped
- 1 large portobello mushroom gills removed, and chopped
- 1/2 oz dried shitake mushrooms rehydrated
- 4 cups low-sodium vegetable broth
- 1 cup frozen peas
- 1/2 tsp dried rosemary

- 1/2 tsp dried thyme
- 1/2 tsp sage
- to taste black pepper
- 1 tbsp dried parsley
- 1 small potato sliced very thin

Instructions

1. Rehydrate the dried shiitake mushrooms according to the package.
2. Preheat the oven to 425 degrees F.
3. In a large pot sauté the onion, shallot, celery, carrots, and garlic in a small amount of water or broth for 5 minutes or until the vegetables are soft. Stir in the diced potato and let cook for 3 minutes.
4. Add the 4 cups of vegetable broth, and then turn heat down to medium heat. Add the peas, herbs and all the mushrooms in the pot and continue cooking on medium-low heat for another 5 minutes, stirring occasionally.
5. Divide mixture into oven-proof bowls. Top the mixture with your chosen topping. Here we are using the potato that is thinly sliced. Place the thin slices on

top of the vegetable mixture. Cook in the oven for 15 minutes.

6. Toppings can include puff pastry, pie pastry, thinly sliced white potatoes, thinly sliced sweet potatoes, thinly sliced carrots and even brussel sprout leaves (steam individual leaves first before layering on top of pie).

12. Spicy Veggie Ramen

Prep Time: 15 Minutes

Cook Time: 25 Minutes

Servings: 2

Ingredients

- 2 cloves garlic chopped
- 3" thumb ginger approximately 2 tbsp
- 1/2 medium onion sliced
- 2 cups low-sodium vegetable broth plus extra for sauté
- 1 tbsp soy sauce
- 4 oz mushroom any variety, sliced
- 2 tsp white or yellow miso
- 2 oz dry ramen noodles
- 2 green onions sliced
- 1 tbsp sriracha or to your taste
- 1 head bok choy with leaves separated
- 1/2 medium carrot or about 1/4 cup grated carrot
- 1 tbsp tomato paste optional

Instructions

1. In a pan heat 1 Tbsp of veggie broth and sauté the onion and garlic for 3 minutes.
2. Add the mushrooms and additional broth as needed. Sauté for 5 more minutes until onions and mushrooms start to carmelize.
3. Add the ginger, broth, soy sauce, miso, green onions, and sriracha. Cook for 1 minutes. If using the tomato paste, add it now.
4. Cook the ramen noodles according to the package.
5. Meanwhile, add the bok choy to the soup and let the bok choy wilt.
6. Once noodles are cooked, drain them and place the noodles in a bowl. Pour the soup over the noodles and top with grated carrots and enjoy!
7. Increase or decrease the sriracha to your taste.

13. Black Bean Corn and Couscous Salad

Prep Time: 30 Minutes

Cook Time: 55 Minutes

Servings: 2

Ingredients

- 1 can black beans drained
- 1 cup frozen corn thawed
- 10 cherry tomatoes halved
- 1/2 green, orange or yellow bell pepper diced
- 1/4 cup cilantro chopped
- 2 cups cooked couscous
- 1/4 cup rice wine vinegar
- 1 tsp Dijon mustard
- 1 clove garlic minced
- to taste black pepper
- 1/2 head Romaine lettuce cut into ribbons or chopped

Instructions

1. In a large bow, combine beans, corn, tomatoes, bell pepper, coriander and couscous.

2. In a small bowl, or jar, mix the vinegar, mustard, garlic and black pepper to make the dressing.

3. Pour the dressing over the salad and toss thoroughly.

4. On a serving plate spread out the romaine lettuce and top with salad.

5. Quinoa instead of couscous

6. Fresh parsley and basil instead of coriander

7. For a sharper taste use balsamic vinegar instead of rice wine vinegar

14. Lentil Burger with Sweet Potato Sticks

Prep Time: 20 Minutes

Cook Time: 40 Minutes

Servings: 2

Ingredients

- 2 cups cooked brown or green lentils
- 1 medium onion finely chopped
- 2 cloves garlic minced
- 1 cup mushrooms (any variety) chopped
- 1 medium beet chopped
- 2 tbsp cilantro leaves freshly chopped
- 3 tbsp parsley leaves freshly chopped
- 1/4 tsp black pepper
- 1 tsp dried ground thyme
- 2 tbsp chia seeds
- 1 1/2 tsp smoked paprika

Extras:

- 4 large leaves outer Romaine lettuce
- 1 medium onion sliced
- 1 large tomato sliced
- 2 large sweet potatoes cut into sticks (or fry shape)

Instructions

1. In a food processor add all the burger ingredients. Process on high or pulse until all the ingredients are mixed well.
2. Make 4 patties and place on a lined baking sheet. Place in the fridge for 15 to 30 minutes. Meanwhile, preheat the oven to Bake at 425°F.
3. Once the burgers are firm, remove from the fridge and cook in the preheated oven for 30 minutes. Check at 15 minutes and flip the burgers. Cook for another 10 to 15 minutes.
4. Cook the sweet potato sticks in the oven at the same time as the burgers. Flip the potato half way through cooking.
5. While the burgers are cooking, prepare the extras. Use the lettuce as a wrap for the burger. The onion and

tomato can be placed on top of the burger before wrapping it.

6. If appropriate with your meal plan, you can use a bun and other condiments.

7. For variety, this recipe can be cooked as a loaf. Once the burger ingredients are combined, pack the mixture into a lined loaf pan and bake in a 400°F oven for 30 minutes. Slice and serve.

15. Piled High Veggie Potato Nachos

Prep Time: 25 Minutes

Cook Time: 55 Minutes

Servings: 1

Ingredients

- 1 medium Russet potato thinly sliced
- 1 serving vegan cheese sauce (see recipe below)
- pinch black pepper
- 1 small scallion chopped
- 1/2 cup low sodium black beans
- 1/2 cup corn fresh or frozen
- 1/2 medium green pepper chopped
- 2 large leaves romaine lettuce shredded
- 2 tbsp sliced black olives
- 2 tbsp cilantro chopped
- 1 tsp chili powder
- 1 medium tomato chopped

Vegan Cheese Sauce

- 1 medium Yukon Gold potato

- 1 medium carrot chopped
- 1/2 cup cashews
- 4 tbsp nutritional yeast
- 1 tsp onion powder
- 2 tsp garlic powder
- 1 tbsp lemon juice
- 1 tsp smoked paprika
- 2 cups hot water (or cooking water from the potato and carrots)

Instructions

1. Preheat the oven to Bake at 400°F. Prepare a baking sheet with parchment paper or silicone mat.
2. Place the potato slices on the prepared baking sheet. Ensure that the potatoes are laid out in a single layer. Cook for 15 minutes or until the potatoes are cooked and browned slightly.
3. Heat up one serving of cheese sauce (see instructions below).
4. Combine the tomatoes, chili powder, cilantro, black pepper and scallion and set aside.
5. Assemble the nachos: on a plate place the potatoes and top with black beans, corn, green pepper, lettuce, black olives, and tomato mixture and serve with a side

of the heated cheese sauce or pour the sauce over the nachos.

For the Vegan Cheese Sauce

1. In a pot of boiling water, cook the potatoes and carrots until soft.
2. Put all the ingredients in a high-speed blender and blend until smooth. Add more water one tablespoon at a time until you get the consistency you wish.
3. Put the unused sauce in an air-tight container and store in the refrigerator.
4. You can add or replace any vegetable you wish to this dish.

16. Thai Jackfruit with Rice

Prep Time: 30 Minutes

Cook Time: 30 Minutes

Servings: 2

Ingredients

- 2 cups fresh jackfruit cut into 1/2" cubes
- 2 tbsp fresh parsley chopped
- 1 lime juice
- 1 tbsp white wine vinegar
- 1 tbsp maple syrup
- 1 tsp low-sodium soy sauce
- 1 tbsp ginger minced
- 1 clove garlic minced
- 1 Thai chili pepper deseeded and finely chopped
- 2 cups cauliflower cut into pieces
- 2 cups brussels sprouts cut in half
- 2 cups brown rice cooked
- 2 tbsp fresh cilantro chopped

Instructions

1. In a bowl mix the parsley, lime juice, white wine vinegar, maple syrup, soy sodium, minced ginger, garlic and chili pepper.
2. Add the prepared jackfruit pieces to the bowl and marinade for 30 minutes or longer.
3. In the meantime, prepare the cauliflower and brussels sprouts.
4. Preheat the oven to Bake at 350°F.
5. In a casserole dish, place the prepared vegetables. Add the marinated jackfruit and juices and mix
6. Cook for 20 to 30 minutes or until vegetables have softened.
7. Serve the jackfruit mixture on a bed of cooked brown rice and top with cilantro.
8. If you wish you can put the jackfruit, cauliflower and brussels sprouts on a skewer and cook on a grill. Remember to soak the skewers in water for 15 minutes before putting the vegetables on the skewers.

17. Asian Grain Bowl

Prep Time: 25 Minutes

Cook Time: 55 Minutes

Servings: 1

Ingredients

- 1 cup brown rice cooked
- 1 sheet Nori
- 1/2 tbsp rice vinegar
- 1/2 cup edamame
- 1/2 cup water chestnuts sliced
- 1/2 cup bean sprouts
- 1 stalk green onion
- 1 carrot cut into matchsticks
- 1/2 cucumber cubed
- 2 cups bok choy leaves separated
- 1/2 cup tofu mashed
- 1/2 tbsp sriracha

Instructions

1. Place the cooked brown rice into the center of a large bowl.
2. Surround the rice with each of the ingredients in clusters.
3. Mash tofu with a fork and mix in the sriracha. Add to the center of the bowl or use as a dip.
4. You can put any vegetables into this bowl such as celery, bamboo shoots, and napa cabbage.

18. Potato Curry with Spinach

Prep Time: 10 Minutes

Cook Time: 30 Minutes

Servings: 2

Ingredients

- 4 medium potatoes (about 1 lb) peeled and chopped into 1" chunks
- 1 tbsp low-sodium vegetable broth
- 1 medium onion finely chopped
- 2 cloves garlic minced
- 2 tsp ginger finely chopped
- 1/2 tsp cumin seeds
- 2 medium tomatoes chopped
- 1 tsp curry powder
- 1/2 tsp black pepper or to taste
- 1/2 cup thick coconut milk
- 6 cups baby spinach

Instructions

1. Cut the peeled potatoes into 1" chunks and place in a saucepan with cold water. Bring to a boil and cook until just barely tender, about 15 to 20 minutes. Ensure that you don't over cook the potatoes.
2. Heat the vegetable broth in a large frying pan over medium heat. Add onion, garlic, ginger and cumin. Cook, stirring frequently, until the onion is soft. Add tomatoes, curry powder; reduce the heat and cover. Cook, stirring occasionally until tomatoes have softened.
3. Add potatoes to pan, Cook, with lid on, stirring occasionally until potatoes are hot. The mixture should now have a stew consistency. If more liquid is needed add a little bit of water.
4. Stir in pepper and coconut milk.
5. Add the spinach and cover for a few minutes so the spinach can wilt. Serve.
6. Instead of spinach used sweet chard, collard greens or bok choy.

19. Vegetable Chipotle Chili with Quinoa

Prep Time: 10 Minutes

Cook Time: 30 Minutes

Servings: 2

Ingredients

- 1 cup uncooked quinoa
- 1 clove garlic minced
- 1 medium onion chopped
- 2 - 3 medium oyster mushrooms chopped
- 2 tbsp water or vegetable broth used for sautéing vegetables
- 1 small to medium bytternut squash peeled and chopped
- 19 oz can black beans drained and rinsed
- 1 large carrot peeled and chopped
- 28 oz can whole tomatoes with juice
- 2 tbsp chipotle powder
- 1/2 tsp pepper
- 1 tbsp cacao powder
- 1 medium zucchini chopped

- 1 cup favorite fresh greens (spinach, arugula, mixed greens, etc.)

Instructions

1. Cook quinoa in 1 1/2 cups of water or broth. Cook for 15 minutes on medium heat. Remove from heat and let it sit covered for 5 minutes.
2. Meanwhile, sauté onion, garlic, and mushrooms in 2 tbsp broth until onions are translucent, approximately 5 minutes.
3. Add butternut squash, carrot, beans, tomatoes, chipotle powder, cacao powder, pepper and bring to a boil then simmer for 30 minutes until squash and carrots are soft. Adjust the spices to your taste.
4. Add the zucchini and simmer for an additional 5 minutes.
5. Serve chili over the quinoa and serve with fresh greens such as spinach.

20. 3 Bean Chili

Prep Time: 10 Minutes

Cook Time: 45 Minutes

Servings: 6

Ingredients

- 1/4 cup Vegetable Broth, Low-Sodium
- 3 cup Onion
- 6 Cloves Garlic
- 1 Green Bell Pepper
- 1 Red Bell Pepper
- 1 tbsp Chili Powder
- 2 tbsp Ground Cumin
- 1/4 tsp Oregano
- 1 1/2 tsp Sweet Paprika
- 3 cup Pinto Beans (Cooked)
- 3 cup Red Kidney Beans (Cooked)
- 3 cup Black Beans (Cooked)
- 3 cup Canned Diced Tomatoes, Low-Sodium
- 1/2 cup Tomato Paste
- 1/2 cup Canned Green Chili

- 2 cup Water
- 1/2 tsp Ground Black Pepper

Instructions

1. In a large saucepan over medium heat, heat up the vegetable broth. Add the onion, green and red bell pepper, and garlic. Sauté, stirring until the onions are soft, 5 to 7 minutes.
2. Add the seasonings, all beans, diced tomatoes, tomato, green chilis, and water.
3. Bring to a boil, reduce heat and simmer for 30 to 40 minutes.
4. Serve in bowls.
5. Add more water if needed to achieve the consistency you prefer.

21. Barley and Kale Bowl

Prep Time: 15 Minutes

Cook Time: 15 Minutes

Servings:

Ingredients

- 1 cup Hulled Barley
- 1 tbsp Cilantro
- 1/2 cup Pinto Beans
- 4 cup Kale
- 1 cup Yellow Pepper
- 1/2 cup Cucumber,
- 1 cup Cherry Tomatoes
- 1/2 cup Carrot
- 1/4 cup Lime Juice
- 1 tsp Lime Zest
- 1/2 tsp Mexican Spice Blend

Instructions

1. Mix cilantro and pinto beans with the cooked barley.
2. Prepare the kale, bell pepper, cucumber, tomatoes, and carrots.
3. Prepare the dressing by mixing the lime juice, lime zest, and Mexican spice. Set aside.
4. In a large serving bowl layer the chopped kale on the bottom then top in sections with the cucumbers, carrots, tomatoes and pepper leaving space for the barley mixture.
5. Scoop the barley mixture into its own section on top of kale.
6. Drizzle the lime dressing on top and sprinkle with the lime zest.
7. Alternate spices could be sumac, cumin, curry.
8. Instead of pinto use your favorite beans such as black or red kidney beans

22. Sweet Potato Bruschetta

Prep Time: 15 Minutes

Cook Time: 25 Minutes

Servings: 1

Ingredients

- 2 cup Sweet Potato
- 1 tsp Garlic Powder
- 3 cup Heirloom Cherry Tomatoes
- 1/4 cup Red Onion
- 1/4 cup White Onion
- 1/2 cup Fresh Basil
- 2 tbsp Fresh Cilantro
- 3 Cloves Garlic
- 1 tbsp Balsamic Vinegar
- 1/2 tsp Black Pepper

Instructions

1. Preheat the oven to 400°F.

2. Scrub the sweet potato. No need to remove skin unless you wish to. Slice the potato lengthwise about ½-inch so you have bread-like slices.You should have 3 or 4 slices. Or you can slice them into ½ inch coins, whichever you prefer.

3. Rub each slice with garlic powder and place the potato slices on a lined baking sheet. Bake for 30 minutes or until the potato is cooked but still firm.

4. Meanwhile mix all the remaining bruschetta ingredients together and set aside to allow the flavors to mix.

5. Once cooked remove the potatoes from the oven and place on a plate. Top with the tomato bruschetta and enjoy.

6. Instead of sweet potato use russet potato, portobello mushroom.

23. Bok Choy Wild Mushroom Soba Noodle Soup

Prep Time: 15 Minutes

Cook Time: 20 Minutes

Servings: 2

Ingredients

- 4 cup Shiitake Mushrooms
- 1/2 cup Onion or Shallot
- 2 tbsp Fresh Ginger
- 6 Garlic Cloves
- 2 tbsp Coconut Aminos
- 8 cup Vegetable Broth
- 1 cup Green Peas
- 1 cup Soba Noodles
- 8 cup Baby Bok Choy
- 2 cup Carrots
- 1/2 cup Green Onions
- 2 tbsp Dry Toasted Sesame Seeds

Instructions

1. In a small amount of water, cook the sliced onions until they are translucent in color

2. Add the mushrooms and cook them for about 5 minutes.

3. Stir in the fresh ginger and garlic then cook until fragrant.

4. Add the coconut aminos and stir, cook until the mushrooms release water.

5. Stir in the vegetable broth and bring the mixture to a boil.

6. Add the green peas, noodles, and bok choy leaves. Cook until noodles are tender for about 5 to 6 minutes.

7. In the meantime, dry toast the sesame seeds in a small pan. Make sure you watch the seeds so they don't burn. Toast them until they are nice and golden.

8. Ladle into a bowl and top with the carrots, green onions, and sesame seeds.

9. You can use whatever mushrooms that you prefer.

24. Asparagus Cucumber Onion Salad with Beans

Prep Time: 20 Minutes

Cook Time: 55 Minutes

Servings: 2

Ingredients

- 1 cup fresh asparagus (white, green, or a mixture) cut in 2" pieces
- 1 medium English cucumber thinly sliced
- 2 medium scallions (or green onions) sliced on a diagonal
- 1/4 cup cilantro chopped
- 1 head Boston lettuce
- 1 1/2 cup chickpeas
- 1 1/2 tbsp rice vinegar
- 1 1/2 tsp low-sodium soy sauce
- 1 lemon's juice
- 1 tbsp fresh chives chopped

Instructions

1. For the dressing mix together the rice vinegar, soy sauce and lemon juice and set aside.
2. In a large bowl combine the asparagus, cucumber, scallion, cilantro, chickpeas and lettuce.
3. Pour the dressing over the vegetable mixture and mix well.
4. Top with chives.
5. Instead of chickpeas add your favorite beans.

25. Butternut Buddha Bowl with Black Beans

Prep Time: 12Minutes

Cook Time: 5 Minutes

Servings: 2

Ingredients

- 8 cup Spinach or Other Greens
- 4 cup Butternut Squash
- 2 cup Apple
- 1 cup Corn
- 1 cup Black Beans
- 1 tbsp Fresh Ginger
- 4 tbsp Apple Cider Vinegar
- 2 tsp Black Pepper
- 4 tsp Curry Powder

Instructions

1. Place the greens at the bottom of the bowl.

2. Cut the butternut squash in half and remove the seeds. Finely chop.

3. Steam butternut squash until soft, about 8-10 minutes.

4. Chop the apple, drain the beans, and thaw the corn.

5. Peel and grate or chop your ginger.

6. Assemble all the ingredients over the bed of greens.

7. Add the apple cider vinegar, black pepper, and curry powder.

8. Toss well to combine all flavors together.

9. Feel free to substitute a whole grain such as quinoa or buckwheat for the corn in this recipe.

26. Easy Homemade Potato Chips

Prep Time: 15Minutes

Cook Time: 20 Minutes

Servings: 2

Ingredients

- 1 Large Russet Potato
- 1 tbsp Garlic Powder
- 1 tbsp Onion Powder

Instructions

1. Clean the potato(es). Place into a bowl of water to keep from browning if needed.
2. Place a piece of parchment paper on a large plate.
3. Using a mandoline slicer or other tool, thinly slice the potatoes (set for ⅛" or the thinnest mandoline setting).
4. Place the potatoes in a single layer, ensure they do not overlap, on top of the parchment paper on the plate.

5. Sprinkle garlic and onion powder over the potato slices until they are lightly coated.

6. Cook the potatoes in the microwave on high power for 4-5 minutes.

7. When done cooking, remove the chips and place them in a basket.

8. Repeat this process until all potato slices are cooked.

9. Enjoy your delicious homemade oil-free potato chips!

10. Parchment paper is important to prevent sticking to the plate. Do not place metal in the microwave!

11. Cook time will vary depending on your type of microwave. When trying this recipe for the first time, set the cooking time for 5 minutes and watch the potato slices closely.

12. The potatoes are done cooking when they turn golden brown. Some microwaves will take more time (upwards of 10 minutes), so just keep adding to the cooking time without allowing the microwave to turn off to find out your microwave's specific cooking time successfully.

27. Roasted Red Pepper Potato Bowl

Prep Time: 10Minutes

Cook Time: 45 Minutes

Servings: 2

Ingredients

- 3 cup Sweet Potato
- 1 cup Red Bell Pepper
- 1 cup White Onion
- 6 cup Mixed Greens
- 2 tsp Cinnamon
- 2 tbsp Hemp Seeds
- 2 tbsp Raisins

Instructions

1. Preheat the oven to 450°F.
2. Wash and chop the sweet potato, red bell pepper, and white onion into small even pieces. Roast in the oven for 45 minutes.

3. Meanwhile, place the greens in a large bowl.

4. When the sweet potatoes are soft, the vegetables are done roasting. Place them over the bed of greens.

5. Sprinkle cinnamon, hemp seeds, and raisins on top of your bowl, and enjoy!

6. Refrigerate leftovers in an air-tight container for up to 5 days.

28. Roasted Potato and Asparagus Bowl

Prep Time: 15 Minutes

Cook Time: 45 Minutes

Servings: 2

Ingredients

- 1 cup Red Onion
- 4 cup Yellow Potatoes
- 3 cup Orange Bell Pepper
- 3 cup Asparagus
- 2 tsp Onion Powder
- 2 tsp Garlic Powder
- 2 tbsp Nutritional Yeast
- 4 cup Arugula

Instructions

1. Preheat oven to 450°F. Line a baking sheet with parchment paper or foil.
2. Wash all vegetables. Dice the red onion. Chop potatoes into small bite-size pieces. Cut the center

stem out of bell pepper and then chop into medium-sized pieces. Cut an inch off the base of the asparagus and then chop into small pieces.

3. Toss vegetables with onion powder, garlic powder, and nutritional yeast then place on the baking sheet.

4. Bake for 45 minutes or until potatoes are crispy and the other vegetables are soft.

5. Place arugula in a bowl and top with roasted vegetables. Enjoy!

6. You may use any type of bell pepper that you enjoy for this recipe.

29. Beet Onion Bulgur Bowl

Prep Time: 15 Minutes

Cook Time: 45 Minutes

Servings: 2

Ingredients

- 2 medium raw beets thinly sliced
- 1 small onion thinly sliced into rings
- 1 cup bulgur cooked
- 1 medium carrot grated or spiralized
- 1 stalk celery chopped
- 1/2 cup kidney beans
- 1 cup kale finely chopped
- 1 tbsp dry toasted sesame seeds
- 1 lemon, juiced
- 1 tbsp cilantro finely chopped
- 1/4 tsp paprika regular or smoked (optional)

Instructions

1. Place the first seven ingredients (beets through to kale) in a bowl.

2. Sprinkle the top with toasted sesame seeds, lemon juice, cilantro and paprika on top.

3. Mix together before eating.

4. To cut down the prep time prepare the bulgur ahead. Instead of bulgur use any grain you desire.

30. Zucchini Noodles with Mango Tomato Sauce

Prep Time: 30 Minutes

Cook Time: 35 Minutes

Servings: 2

Ingredients

- 4 cup Zucchini Noodles
- 4 cup Red Tomatoes, chopped
- 1 cup Mango
- 5 Garlic Cloves
- 1 cup White Onion
- 1/2 cup Basil
- 1/4 tsp Black Pepper

Instructions

1. Spiralize or shred zucchini with a mandolin slicer.

2. Prepare the mango tomato sauce by blending tomato, mango, garlic cloves, white onion, basil, and black pepper. Add to the bowl.

3. Slice the mushrooms.

4. Arrange zucchini noodles and beans on a bed of greens.

5. Toss gently to mix and combine flavors.

6. No Zucchini: Use any other type of noodle that you enjoy, yellow squash, sweet potato, carrots, cucumber, beets, or even broccoli stems!